Weight Loss For Women Over 50

Look and Feel Fabulous in 30 Days or Less!

Easy to Follow Diet and Exercise Plan for Women Over 50!

Table of Contents

Introduction

I want to thank you and congratulate you for downloading the book "Weight Loss for Women over 50: Look and Feel Fabulous in 30 Days or Less! Easy to Follow Diet and Exercise Plan for Women Over 50!"

This book contains proven steps and strategies on how to achieve a younger, sexier, healthier, and more energetic you in 30 days or less.

This book will give you information on how to improve yourself. The good news is the information presented herein is based on health facts. There will be no tricks or temporary results promised here. Hopefully, this will be the jumpstart you need to live the rest of your life in a healthier way.

Thanks again for downloading this book, I hope you enjoy it!

responsibility or blame be held against the publisher for any reparation, damages, or monetary loss due to the information herein, either directly or indirectly.

Chapter 1 – Clean Your Life

As mentioned in the introduction, this book is about health, not a temporary fix to look great for your next special occasion. If your goal is the latter, then you are better off buying slimming undergarments to hide your flaws. However, if you are sick of temporary results and really want to make a change in your life, then you must really commit to change. Otherwise, you are only fooling yourself.

Once you *really* decide to improve yourself, the first step is to clean out your lifestyle of junk. Junk includes everything that is unhealthy like too many sweets, processed foods and alcohol, and too much partying, overtime at work and too little sleep. Otherwise, even if you try to maintain a healthier diet and exercise regularly, your unhealthy junk might just cancel out your good results.

Since everyone's lives are different, it will be up to you to determine how to go about making those changes. For example, if your daily schedule leaves little time for exercise, there is really no way to solve this predicament except to make time for exercise. This can mean waking up earlier, spending less time at work, or less time with your friends.

Either way, you have freed up some of your time for exercise.

Since you are already in your 50s and may be set in your ways, it might be difficult to change your ingrained habits, but this need not be the case for you. Most of the time, change is difficult because you are not clear about your goals. That is why the word "really" is emphasized above. The human body is subject to the laws of the natural world. There is no such thing as magic when it comes to health. If anyone tries to make you think so, they are only selling temporary results. Thus, you must realize early on that if you *really* want change, then you must change.

Chapter 2 – The Importance of a Healthy Diet

You will accept a diet plan more readily if you understand how it works. Most people already know the basics of what a healthy diet contains. For example, nobody in her right mind will say that potato chips are as healthy as raw carrot sticks. However, too many people, men and women alike, don't understand how diet ties in with health, and how weight loss is more a matter of health than of calories. This chapter will explain everything.

Most people only start eating more

healthily once they reach their late 20s or early 30s because that's the time when the body starts to degrade after years of eating junk. Those in their teenage years and early 20s can get away with a bad diet because their bodies are more able to regenerate properly even with only a minimal amount of nutrients, but this is only true if they were fed a nutritious diet during their childhood. Nowadays, since more and more parents are feeding their children fast food or processed food, it is no longer uncommon for a child to be obese, for a teenager to have type-II diabetes and for a 20 year old to have a heart attack.

The human body's ability to regenerate and remain healthy is generally based on *both* age and nutrition. Even a young body, like that of a child or a teenager, will soon break down if proper nutrition is not provided. However, if a teenager and a woman in her 50s are both fed the same unhealthy diet, the latter will break down faster due to her age.

Thus, those in their 50s and above must be doubly careful about their diet. If you have not fed yourself properly during your younger years, there is more damage to deal with, so it might take longer – or it might even be unlikely – for your body to be in tip-top shape through proper nutrition alone. For example, if you already suffer from high blood pressure, high cholesterol and the like, it might be advisable to take prescription medication to keep them in control. Otherwise, if you have taken care of yourself or your health condition is not that bad, a healthy diet may be enough to bring your body back to health.

Whether you are taking maintenance medication or not, here is the truth about nutrition for women in their 50s: if you have been following a healthy diet during most of your adult life and have a sufficiently active lifestyle, you don't need to make too many changes. A lot of people think that nutritional needs drastically change for older adults, but that is not true. Once a woman has stopped growing (i.e. she has reached the height Mother Nature has intended for her), then she has technically reached adulthood. From that age on, her nutritional needs will remain relatively stable except during special times like pregnancy, lactation, and illness (Nutritional needs also change for those with physically demanding lives like athletes, but only because they subject their bodies to extreme stress.).

For example, an adult woman's calcium needs remain at 1000 mg until the age of 50 then from 51 onwards, it increases to 1200 mg. The added 200 mg can be easily provided by an extra ounce of cheese daily to an already healthy diet. There is no need to go all out and drink an extra pint of milk or take extra calcium supplements unless your current diet is already deficient in calcium. The slight increase is partly due to the body's decreasing ability to absorb nutrients properly and partly due to the body's decreased ability to regenerate properly. Both are natural consequences of aging. The increased nutritional needs for mature women will be discussed further in chapter 4.

The only reasons why you need to make major changes in your diet as you grow older are if you are already on a very unhealthy one, if you are suffering from one of the many lifestyle diseases, and if you refuse to exercise regularly. To explain, let us consider each separately.

First, regarding being on an unhealthy diet: as explained earlier, the older your body is, the less efficient it is in regenerating itself. Thus, the older you are the more imperative it is for you to avoid an excess of the so-called 'bad' foods.

For example, consuming too much fatty bacon is bad for anyone *regardless* of age, but since younger bodies are more efficient in regenerating themselves, younger people can consume fatty bacon more often without experiencing too many adverse effects. In contrast, since older bodies are less efficient in regenerating themselves, the bad effects of fatty bacon will manifest more easily.

In other words, everyone regardless of age needs to maintain a healthy diet, but this need becomes more imperative with age.

Second, if you are already suffering from a lifestyle disease: obviously, you need to make the necessary changes to avoid making your condition worse. For example, if you suffer from high blood pressure, it may be necessary for you to go on a low-sodium diet. Your doctor is more qualified to tell you what sort of changes you must make.

Third, regarding your refusal to exercise regularly: your level of physical activity affects three things, namely, daily calorie needs, lean muscle mass, and bone mass. Everybody already knows that the more you move, the more calories you need, and the more calories you need the more food you must eat. If you insist on living a sedentary lifestyle, you must consume only a minimum number of calories depending on your ideal weight, otherwise you will get fat.

For example, if your height is 5'3", for a woman, your ideal weight is 115-125 pounds (There will be differences due to build.). The daily calorie need of a sedentary woman is the number of her ideal weight with a 0 added to the end multiplied by 1.2. Hence, if you weigh 120 pounds, then the formula is this: 1200 x 1.2 = 1440.

Eating 1440 calories daily sounds like quite a challenge but it isn't. A usual breakfast of 2 slices of bread with a pat of butter, a cup of whole milk, a large orange and 2 large fried eggs already contains around 600 calories. You can save about 200 calories by omitting the butter, drinking skim milk and poaching the eggs, but the point here is calories can easily add up and the only way to prevent them from adding up is to limit your food consumption.

That might sound like a good idea, and indeed you may have already done this before whenever you wished to lose weight. However, the less food you eat, the less nutrients your body receives. That is why nutritionists advise those on a low-calorie diet, i.e. 500 less calories daily than their normal needs, to take supplements. Thus, if you insist on not exercising and choose to maintain your weight on a low-calorie diet, you must take a nutritional supplement even if your diet is already a healthy one.

However, the older you get, the harder it will be to maintain your ideal weight on a low-calorie diet alone. It is a natural part of the aging process for the body to decrease muscle mass and increase fat mass. The less muscle mass you have, the less calories you need daily because muscle requires more calories to remain alive compared to other cells like fat and bone.

Hence, if currently your weight remains stable on a 1440-calorie diet, in five years, you may find yourself gaining weight because your calorie needs may have dropped to 1300 or less due to muscle loss. You can prevent weight gain by increasing your physical activity or by decreasing your calorie intake; but remember that the less food you eat, the fewer nutrients you can consume from food alone. As your daily calorie requirement drops, even a supplement may not be enough to provide all your nutritional needs. Also, less food results in a less enjoyable life.

You will soon have to choose between eating for your health's sake or for the sake of maintaining your ideal weight. Ironically, maintaining your ideal weight is also necessary for your health. So what's a woman to do?

These problems will all be solved once

you finally accept that exercise is necessary both for weight loss and for your health. Increasing physical activity will not only raise your daily calorie needs, it will also force your body to maintain your current muscle mass and even increase it, thus preventing the decrease in daily calorie needs. Further, it will prevent bone loss which naturally happens during the aging process. This will be discussed further in the next chapter.

Chapter 3 – The Importance of Exercising Properly

The most important benefit of exercise is not weight loss but the overall well-being of your body. Regular exercise keeps the body strong, helps to reduce stress, and has been shown to slow down the effects of aging. Recall that loss of muscle mass is a natural consequence of aging and that exercise helps to prevent this.

Actually, most of the natural consequences of aging like the general weakening of the body and of the immune system, and the loss of bone mass can be prevented with regular exercise. A person who has been active most of her life can maintain the body of a 20 year old despite having a 60 or even 70 year old soul.

That being said, exercise cannot prevent the slowing down of the body's ability to regenerate itself. A physically fit 60-year-old may outrun an out-of-shape 30 year old, but not a physically fit one. Generally speaking, at the age of 40, the body starts to weaken no matter how physically fit it is. In a sport contest between a 20 year old and a 40 year old, if they have similar levels of physical fitness, the 20 year old will always have the advantage. Of course, there are some people in their 40s and 50s who seem to defy the odds and can still out-perform the younger ones, but they are exceptions. Also, it is more likely that while they can outperform a younger person in one contest, if the challenge involves several succeeding contests, they will likely burn out more quickly.

It is due to the reality of the inevitable slowing down of the body that this chapter is titled "The Importance of Exercising *Properly*." There is no shame in admitting one's age and slowing down appropriately when it comes to exercise.

If you have never exercised before or if

more than a year has passed since you last went to the gym, then you must treat yourself as a beginner. This means you must proceed at a slower rate. Doing more than what your body is used to will cause injury. On the other hand, if you have already been a gym rat all your life, then you must learn to listen to your body to know when it's time to slow down. A safe rule is to start to slow down once you reach the age of 40. Too often older adults only slow down after an injury, but there is no need to wait for that to happen. It's always better to be on the safe side. Remember that you exercise for your health's sake, not to show off to other people.

What does it mean to slow down? It means either doing slower exercises with less impact on the joints, or increasing rest days, or decreasing exercise time, or all of these. Here are some examples of slowing down:

- Brisk walking instead of jogging

- 20 minutes of jogging instead of 40 minutes

- Exercising 3 times a week instead of 5 times

Take note that slowing down will have different meanings depending on your age and physical fitness level. Someone who has been jogging daily for 20 years can slow down to jogging every other day, while someone who has only jogged 3 times a week may slow down to 2 times a week. Whatever the case, slowing down always means decreasing your usual intensity and duration, but not too much that your exercise regime becomes too easy for you. It takes some trial and error to correctly slow down, but a consultation with a professional trainer and/or your doctor may make things easier.

Exercising properly also means doing all the kinds of exercises your body needs. These include aerobic or cardiovascular exercises and strength training exercises. The first involves doing an activity which raises your heart beat to the point when conversation becomes difficult. The intensity, i.e. speed, of the activity will depend on your current level of physical fitness. Beginners will likely find that a brisk 20-minute walk already raises their heart rate, but for the more physically fit they need to move faster by jogging or running. Once an activity no longer makes conversation difficult, you must increase the intensity or else your fitness level will not improve.

Increasing your fitness level is important for two reasons: first, the more fit you are, the healthier and stronger your heart and lungs are. Your risk of heart disease and type-II diabetes decreases and your cholesterol levels will improve. Your body will also be more efficient in its use of energy allowing you to work for longer hours without getting tired.

Second, the more fit you are, the more intense your exercise activities can be, which means you can burn more calories in less time. For example, a beginner can only do a brisk 20 minute walk, perhaps at the speed of 2 mph. This will burn only 100 calories for a 120 pound woman (more or less depending on your height and weight). Since a beginner can only exercise at most 3 times a week or else risk getting injured, that's only a total burn of 300 calories per week. With 3500 calories to burn in order to lose a pound of fat, it's going to take a long time before your extra 10 pounds are burned off.

In contrast, a more physically fit person can jog for 30 minutes at a speed of 4 mph or faster. This will burn about 200-300 calories for a 120-pound woman. Also, a fit person will be able to exercise more frequently, say about 5 times a week. That's a total calorie burn of 1000-1500 calories per week. A pound of fat can be burned in 2-3 weeks.

Aerobic exercise is great for improving

physical fitness and burning calories, but it must be combined with strength training to gain all the possible benefits of regular exercise. Strength training means forcing your muscles to carry more weight than it is used to like carrying dumbbells or doing calisthenics, i.e. body weight exercises, like push-ups. This activity forces your body to create more muscle mass thus preventing or decreasing the inevitable loss of muscle due to aging. This also makes your body build more bone to prevent conditions like osteoporosis.

While aerobic exercise can also help to build more muscle and bone, by itself it is not enough to offset the muscle and bone loss due to aging. People in their 20s and 30s can get away with only doing aerobic exercise because their bodies have not yet begun to lose muscle and bone (which is not to say that they should because they will miss out on the benefits of strength training, like more defined muscles), but more mature adults absolutely need to include strength training in their fitness routine.

Chapter 4 – Putting It All Into Action: Diet

Knowing what you need to do and why will not improve your body if you don't put everything into action. In this chapter, let us consider how to do that exactly starting with your diet.

The best nutritional advice for any age group is the food pyramid. Some people make fun of the food pyramid for being out of fashion, but it is based on solid evidence from years of research by nutritionists and medical professionals. That's more than can be said about the fad diets of recent years like the high-protein diet and the blood type diet.

This is the food pyramid in a nutshell with examples of what a serving looks like:

- 6-11 servings of whole grains, e.g. 1 slice of whole grain bread

- 3-5 servings of vegetables, e.g. ½ cup of cooked vegetables

- 2-3 servings of fruit, e.g. 1 medium orange

- 2-3 servings of *lean* protein, e.g. 8 ounces of chicken without skin

- 2-3 servings of *low-fat or non-fat* dairy or other calcium-rich food, e.g. 8 ounces of low-fat or skim milk

- A small amount of fatty and sugary foods, e.g. a smear of butter, a teaspoon of honey

This is a very general description of a healthy diet. What you must consume will depend on your daily calorie needs and personal preferences. For example, if you are trying to lose weight and must limit your calorie intake, then choose skim milk over low-fat milk. Also, vegetarian protein sources like tofu have fewer calories than animal protein sources. Total servings of whole grains range from 6-11 depending on how active you are. If you are very active but don't need to lose weight, e.g. an athlete, then you must consume 11 servings.

Sedentary people must limit their servings to 6.

Beyond a healthy diet, here are the nutritional extras women in their 50s need:

- *Increase calcium to 1200 mg.* This can easily be achieved by adding an extra 8 ounces of skim milk to your already healthy diet. If you must be strict with your calorie count, extra calcium can be provided by supplements. Increased calcium is necessary to prevent bone loss. While strength training makes the body produce more bone, it cannot do so without calcium.

- *Increase vitamin D to 600 iu.* This vitamin is necessary for the proper absorption of calcium. Fatty fish like tuna are the best sources of vitamin D.

- *Increase vitamin B12 to 2.4 mcg.* Adults over the age of 50 usually start to have difficulty absorbing this vitamin from food sources, so it might be better to take it in the form of a supplement.

- *Increase omega-3 to 500 mg.* Mature adults are at greater risk of heart disease and this nutrient helps to decrease that. If you are already fit and have been living a healthy lifestyle even before you hit your 50s, then there is less need for you to be worried about omega-3; but if you are only starting to pay attention to your health, then it's better to be on the safe side. Serving fatty fish like tuna and salmon twice a week will kill two birds with one stone by providing you with sufficient amounts of omega-3 and vitamin D. Don't worry about the word 'fatty.' The fats in fish are good for you unlike the fats in red meat.

These are the major nutritional changes you need to make once you reach your 50s. Everything else remains the same as for women of a younger age group and can be sufficiently provided by your adequately healthy diet.

There you go! There are no tricks here and no required special exotic foods, only good solid nutritional advice which is backed by years of study. If you eat properly for one month straight, you will notice a difference; and if you maintain this diet forever, you will continue to see improvement.

Since the food pyramid emphasizes lean

protein, low-fat dairy and only a small amount of fats and sugars, you can lose a significant amount of weight through diet alone. For example, a typical Western breakfast of fried eggs and buttered toast is very high in calories, but when you follow the food pyramid, you must limit your consumption of fat. Thus, the eggs must be poached or boiled, and the toast must either be unbuttered or only lightly buttered. Doing this every day will save you at least 200 calories a day, and that's just from breakfast. In 30 days, you can save 6000 calories which means a total loss of 1.7 pounds even without exercise. Remember that this is just from the changes you made in your daily breakfast. If you make further changes in your other meals, and add your calorie burn from exercise, you can easily slash at least 5 pounds off the scale in 30 days or less.

Chapter 5 – Putting It All Into Action: Exercise

In this chapter, let us consider how to put your newfound knowledge about exercise into action.

For complete beginners, start with any low impact and low intensity aerobic activity like walking. As long as it gets your heart rate up to the point when conversation becomes difficult, it can be considered aerobic exercise. During the first two weeks, go extremely slow to avoid injuring your body. Give yourself at least a day's rest in between exercise routines.

For example, on Mondays, Wednesdays, and Fridays, go for a 20-minute walk. You must find the time to do this, but the best time is always in the morning before work. That way, you will get exercise out of the way and you won't find yourself making excuses like being too tired after work.

By the third week, your body will be used to exercise so you can increase the intensity and/or frequency of exercise. Safely increasing intensity and frequency will always depend on trial and error. Listen to your body and dial it down when you feel pain or feel like you might pass out.

As for strength training exercises, there is a higher danger of injury when beginners try to use equipment like dumbbells and barbells for the first time. It is better to ask the help of a professional trainer. Alternatively, simple calisthenics like squats and push-ups can be attempted on your own.

You don't need to hire a professional trainer if you choose to do simple calisthenics, but you must familiarize yourself with the proper form of each exercise. Even relatively simple exercises like squats, while easy to master, can result in injury if done incorrectly.

Find the time to do strength training exercises at least twice a week. If you do aerobic exercises on Mondays, Wednesdays, and Fridays, then you can do strength training on Tuesdays and Thursdays. There is no time limit for these exercises but you must do at least one exercise for each major muscle group. Beginners can give themselves a complete workout by doing at least 10 repetitions each of wall push-ups to work the upper body, crunches to work the abdominals, and squats to work the lower body.

To do a wall push-up, stand before a wall at arm's length then make a small step forward. Place your palms on the wall. Exhale then bend your arms to lower your face towards the wall. Inhale then straighten your arms but don't lock your elbows. This is one repetition.

To do a crunch, lie on the floor with your knees bent and feet flat on the floor. Place your hands behind your head or crossed over your chest. Exhale then lift your upper body off the floor. The movement doesn't have to be high as long as you feel the effort on your abdominal muscles. Try to avoid raising your feet off the floor as you raise your chest. Hold for one second, inhale then lower. This is one repetition.

To do a squat, stand before a chair with your feet slightly apart. Exhale then try to sit but don't allow your butt to touch the chair. Keep your back straight and don't allow your knees to go over your toes. Hold for a second, inhale then stand up. This is one repetition.

For all exercises, NEVER hold your breath. Always breathe as instructed.

If you are a complete beginner to exercise, you cannot reasonably expect to see drastic results after only 30 days. Even so, you will still feel slight benefits like having more energy. If you continue to exercise and make it a life habit, you will gain even more benefits.

Conclusion

Thank you again for downloading this book!

I hope this book was able to help you to know how to improve your health and become a better person in 30 days or less without the gimmicks or tricks. Remember, you're never too old to look and feel fabulous!

The next step is to try out the tips listed here and see what works for you.

Finally, if you enjoyed this book, then I'd like to ask you for a favor, would you be kind enough to leave a review for this book on Amazon? It'd be greatly appreciated!

Thank you and good luck!